A MODERN DAY GUIDE

to

MASSAGE FOR CHILDREN

by Tina Allen

DISCLAIMER

This book contains techniques and massage routines that are designed for toddlers and growing children. The information contained herein is in no way intended to replace medical advice, but rather to offer suggestions on how you might apply nurturing touch for healthy children. These techniques are not advised for use on infants, or children with special healthcare needs, without further professional guidance.

The author does not dispense medical advice or prescribe the use of any technique as form of specific treatment without the advice of a medical professional. A healthcare professional should be consulted prior to beginning any massage program to ensure the health and safety of the child. Neither the author nor the publisher can be held responsible for any damage or injury resulting from the use of the techniques in this book.

BLUE MISO BOOKS
bluemisobooks.com

Printed in China

ISBN 978-1-940279-00-8

Graphic design and Illustration: Amelia Gutierrez.
Editorial design: Luciana Kirszenbaum.

For my son, Otis, husband, Shad and my Dad
for their constant love and support.

FOREWORD

Evolving research continues to show substantial health and emotional benefits from touch, physical nurturance and closeness for everyone from premature infants to the elderly. In the United States our society is more physically isolated than even those in other Western nations such as those in Central and Southern Europe. The rugged individualism and independence that has been formative in our society has also led to the breakdown of extended families and to the development of more emotional and physical isolation.

We shy away from touch and closeness for fear of crossing boundaries. Our fear of bad touch drives our behavior more than our basic need for good touch. This is paradoxical for the fear of bad touch often leads us to a situation where we do not develop the skills to get our needs for closeness, nurturance and tactile stimulation met with good touch.

As a society with many avenues of good touch feared or cut off, what is left is less whole, less healthy touch. It is as if we are a kingdom that taxes its farms and businesses out of existence, then despairs at the lack of food and employment and is surprised to find robbers in the streets.

Tina Allen and her Liddle Kidz foundation are at the leading edge of reintegrating good touch into our society. By teaching the principles and sharing techniques that have been refined over her career in Pediatric Massage, Tina makes learning a foundation of straightforward massage skills something that is accessible to everyone. The knowledge she shares in regard to what works best for each developmental stage is invaluable for professional and parent alike. The techniques and stories are easy to work with and a delight to use.

Tina is a highly committed and truly passionate individual. She shares the techniques and specific skills she has developed and mastered and taught to Neonatologists, Pediatricians and Massage therapists across the globe. Studying this work and incorporating it into your home life or your professional practice can improve the quality of life for your family, your clients, our patients and the world.

Touch is like rain. It is something we have insulated ourselves from in our society to our detriment. Without it, our lives are desiccated, drier and do not reach their full potential. If we can find ways to let it be a regular part of our lives, we can root, grow, and flourish. As we reconnect with our needs for tactile contact and closeness through teaching this foundation to our children, we can look forward to a healthier, happier society of more whole individuals.

Robert D. Sheeler, M.D.
Mayo Clinic

TABLE OF CONTENTS

INTRODUCTION

In this Modern-Day Guide, learn the who, why, when, where and how to provide healthy Massage for Children.

The information contained within this book has been presented to medical professionals, neonatologists, pediatricians, massage therapists and parents around the globe. It is written to be of equal value to both the professional and parent as the material is designed with safety and nurturance as the primary focus.

Children require tactile stimulation through a variety of sources in order to fully develop their body, mind and spirit. Those who receive massage therapy, may experience many benefits, including an awareness of boundaries, stress reduction and an overall sense of well being.

Understandably, children have different physical, emotional and developmental needs than those of adults, which is why this book was written using childhood developmental considerations. Throughout this guide, you will learn the importance of massage and how to use touch therapy to interact with children using age appropriate activities, storytelling, songs and rhymes that provide appropriate stimulation opportunities.

I hope the information shared within these pages will lead you to many hours of sharing safe, nurturing touch with the growing children in your life.

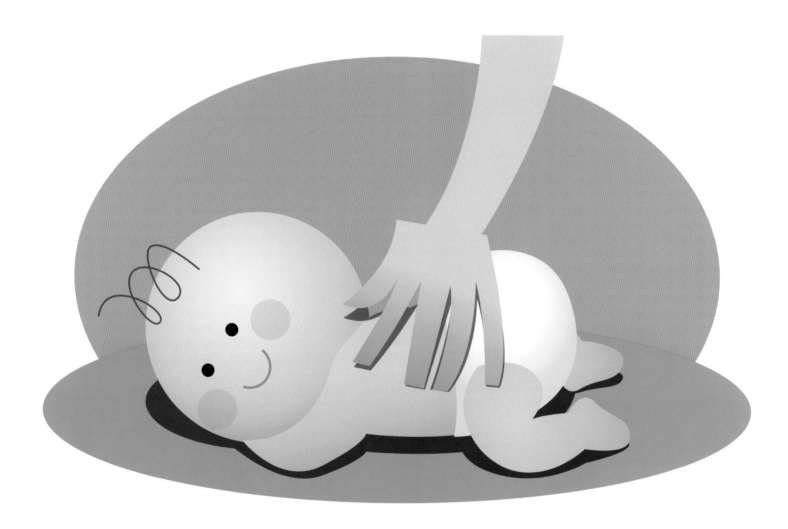

Babies and children simply love to be touched. In fact, they thrive on it, and it is a crucial part of their growth and development.

Touch therapy research has demonstrated that nurturing touch for children is critical in establishing the foundation of their overall sense of well-being. Normal affectionate touching is important, however, a regular routine of massage therapy for a child promotes more integrated physiological, neurological and psychological development and function.

When children experience different forms of touch, they create their own feelings and beliefs about the types of touch they receive. Without appropriate amounts of nurturing touch, they may become susceptible to inappropriate and confusing touch, feel the effects of neglect, and may not develop to reach their full potential. Just as important as a child's physical and cognitive development, their social and emotional development grows based on receiving rich tactile experiences. For children specifically, significant aspects of their emotional development is established through healthy and appropriate touch.

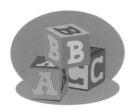

WHY | BENEFITS OF MASSAGE

Massage is an evidence-based, safe and effective way to provide appropriate tactile stimulation to encourage a child's growth and development. While at the same time, it is a fun way to share in a developmentally appropriate activity.

The benefits of massage therapy can be achieved during a relaxing thirty minute full body session, or simply by massaging the hands or feet for a few moments. The greatest benefit is received by the child when the experience is accompanied by nurturing intention, mutual respect and connection.

The physical, psychological and emotional benefits of touch for infants and children have been well documented in published research studies. The evidence that massage provides global benefits to a child's health far outweighs any evidence of negative effects.

Clinical research has shown that massaging a child can help soothe common discomforts, promote restful sleep, and increase healthy attachment and bonding. Studies have reported a variety of behavioral and developmental benefits such as improved immune function, digestion and the healthy development of the white matter portion of the brain.

All children develop and grow at their own rate. So, they may each experience massage therapy differently from one another.

CHILDREN WHO RECEIVE MASSAGE THERAPY MAY EXPERIENCE THE FOLLOWING BENEFITS:
- Decreased anxiety and stress hormones.
- Reduced aggressive behavior.
- Enhanced respiratory function.
- Production of optimal hormone levels.
- Increased body awareness (visual, tactile and proprioceptive input.)
- Improved muscle tone and muscle relaxation.
- Improved joint mobility.
- Reduced hypersensitivity to tactile input.
- Increased quality and quantity of vocalization.
- Enhanced body image and self esteem.
- Increased bonding.
- Increased healthy sense of boundaries.

CHILDREN ARE OUR GREATEST GIFT
AND SHOULD BE TREATED
WITH EXTRAORDINARY CARE!

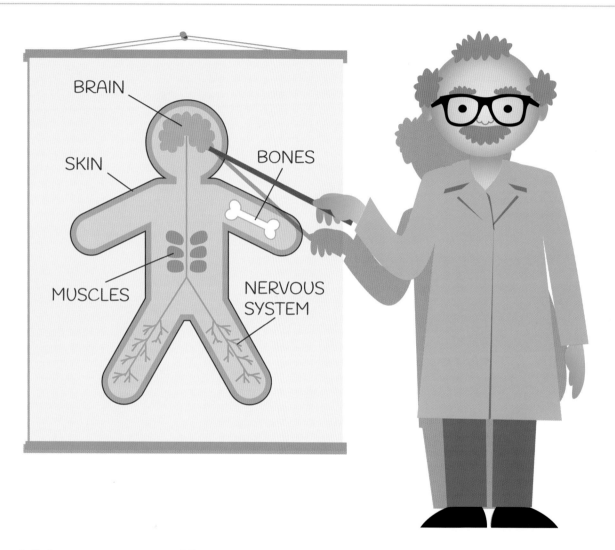

Sure, children may seem like small adults. Let's face it; many of them are even smarter than some of the "grown-ups" we know.

However, the reality is they mature and develop at their own pace. When it comes to using massage and touch therapy, there are some important developmental considerations to keep in mind.

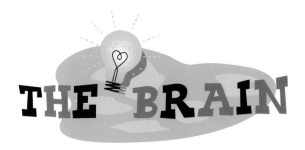

THE BRAIN

At birth, the brain is especially responsive to sensory stimulation which makes up the majority of a baby's learning experiences during the first two years of life. Throughout the first five to seven years of life, a massive amount of brain development occurs. Tactile stimulation, just like any new experience, causes the brain and nervous system to make connections throughout the body.

Many healthcare and education professionals emphasize special importance for brain development during the first three years of life. It is believed that during this time the brain has the greatest potential for learning and developing, but it is critical to understand that providing massage after the first three years may have just as many benefits. Children of all ages experience numerous benefits of massage including more restful sleep, improved immune function and increased body awareness.

Specific massage and movement techniques may help to strengthen a structure in the brain called the Corpus callosum, a thick band of nervous tissue that connects the right and left hemispheres of the brain allowing the right and left sides of the brain to communicate and share information.

Scientists suggest that it is critical to increase the communication between these two hemispheres to improve focus, concentration and for optimum brain growth.

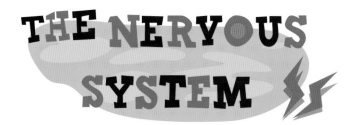

THE NERVOUS SYSTEM

The nervous system controls everything we do and behaves similar to a telephone system. Information is transmitted to and from the brain, via the nervous system, much like sound is carried via telephone lines from one phone to another.

As a child grows, his or her nervous system becomes more mature. Walking, running, balance, coordination, and the range of movement are determined by functioning of this important system.

Most infants learn to crawl before they learn to walk. Some children learn to walk early, while others may take a bit longer. Eventually, the brain starts to create pathways between the neurons, so things become easier and children master the skills to do them better. Once the highest level of neurological functioning is achieved, the child will have the ability to fully react to changes that are happening within their body, and the world around them.

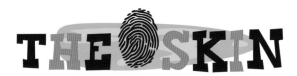

THE SKIN

It is important that we understand some marked differences between the skin of the child and adult.

Though rarely thought of in the same context as the heart or liver, the skin is an organ and has some very important functions. It is responsible for absorption of moisture, temperature regulation, and protection.

The skin is a very sophisticated but underappreciated body system – it keeps the inside in and the outside out. It literally defines the boundary between self and the environment.

Children's skin is more fragile, thinner and softer. It is also more porous and mobile. At earlier stages of development, sensory receptors are not all connected to the central nervous system, which is why young children may not perceive excessive heat, cold or pressure.

Touch can easily cause overstimulation, as children have more tactile receptors per square centimeter, than adults. Most of us have approximately 1,000-5,000 different sensory receptors per square centimeter. These tactile receptors are most compact in the hand, fingertips and lips, so in turn these areas may be more sensitive to touch.

Being that a child is smaller in size, there is less surface area to cover when providing massage.

Therefore your hands will more easily cover a larger percentage of their body surface. This may present the dual risks of heat release from the body and overstimulation. On the other hand, the child has a greater proportion of skin surface area to body size from which the child loses heat. So, they are also at risk for becoming chilled more easily. Temperature control for children is typically not complete until around the age of five.

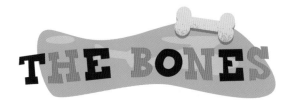

THE BONES

During the fetal stage, the bones start to change from mostly cartilage to more solid bone. When a baby is born, many of their bones are still not calcified, or fused. Many of the bones appear as cartilage and progressively harden during development. Children have 330 bones and adults have 206. This is due to the fact that not all bones are fused at birth. The fusing and calcification (hardening) process takes place over time, with girls typically developing two years faster than boys.

Children's bone growth and development is determined by many factors including; their family genetics implied physiological age, health, nutrition, and environmental factors, such as appropriate stimulation and play. Growth spurts may appear at different times in a child's life and massage may be very helpful during these periods.

Throughout the growth process, children's bones are typically more flexible and porous than adults'. Cartilage growth plates at the ends of all long bones cause bones to grow in length. During childhood, the growth rate is rapid. If a growth plate is injured, it can result in uneven or disrupted growth. Causes of injury, may include trauma, twisting, squeezing, pulling and excessive weight bearing. To help prevent injury, you should use slow sustained pressure, not rapid movements, and be mindful of supporting the joints.

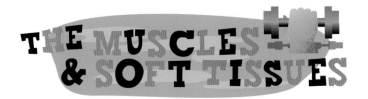

THE MUSCLES & SOFT TISSUES

When you look at an infant, it is obvious their muscles appear softer than an older child's.

Children's muscles are less dense and rigid than an adult's. This means that the pressure applied during massage should not be too firm or deep.

In thinking of the muscles, we should also consider other soft tissues. For children, their periosteum, (a membrane that covers bones containing blood vessels and nerves that provide nourishment), is thicker, and more biologically active.

The tendons and ligaments are less rigid, causing greater range of motion in the joints. This explains why being gentle and learning proper techniques is important to avoid injury to the joints. Injury can be caused if you provide massage directly in those areas or use too much pressure.

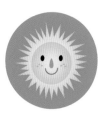

COMMUNICATION

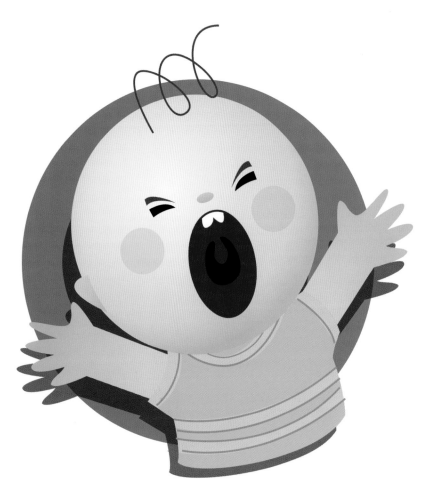

Communication is imperative to providing safe and effective nurturing touch. Some children may not yet be speaking in words that we readily understand, so, paying attention to non-verbal communication is important.

Even with children who are verbal, the non-verbal cues help us understand those words they are not saying out loud. Always watch the child's face and body for signs of discomfort, such as grimacing or tensing of specific areas.

When speaking with a child who is verbal or not, you should use appropriate language and words that will likely be developmentally appropriate.

When introducing nurturing touch to children, it may be beneficial to use names for massage strokes that children can relate to. Use words that may help to describe feelings associated with the types of touch they may receive from each technique, such as hugs, rain and marching.

AGE APPROPRIATE LANGUAGE

TODDLERS | AGES 1 -3 YEARS OLD

- Uses up to 100 words by age 2, 1000 words by age 3.
- Starts to form simple sentences (2 – 2 ½ years).
- Use words that a child may understand "good touch", "safe touch", " "nice touch".

PRESCHOOL | AGES 3 -5 YEARS OLD

- Uses 3-5 word sentences, vocabulary of 900-1500 words.
- Use words that a child may understand to describe massage "gentle touch".
- Explain how massage might feel "your body may feel warm/sleepy".

SCHOOL AGE | AGES 5 -12 YEARS OLD

- 5 year old vocabulary consists of 2100 or more words.
- Ask the child what they think massage is, and use those words (if appropriate) to describe it.
- Explain how massage affects the body.

ADOLESCENT | AGES 12 - 18 YEARS OLD

- Will likely have quite an extensive vocabulary (including words that you wish they wouldn't use).
- Don't talk down to them even a little bit or you may lose their trust completely.

ALL AGES

- Making them feel safe and in control is critical to their enjoyment of the experience.
- Take adequate time to answer any questions respectfully.
- When introducing massage, begin with less contact and less interaction early, building on that as you gain their trust.

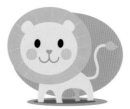

WHEN TO MASSAGE

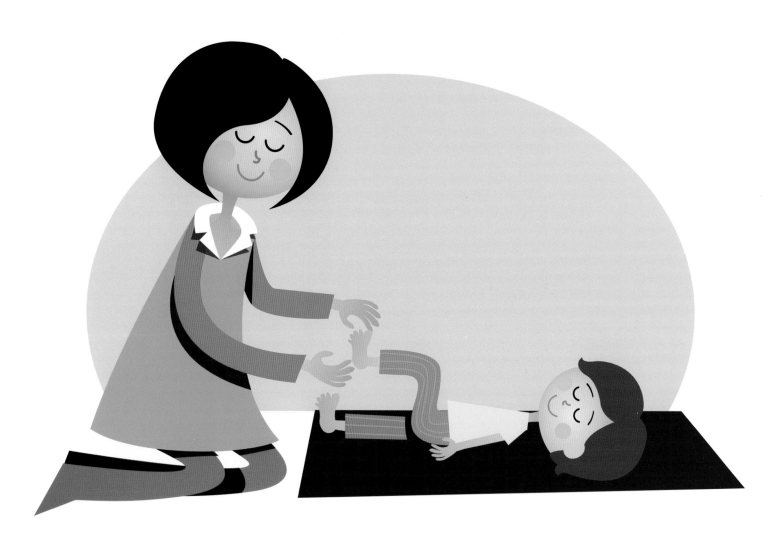

Massage is appropriate for children at any time they request it, or give permission to receive touch therapy.

It should be a time when you have the ability to take a moment to relax prior to beginning. Providing massage when you are not relaxed may only lead to more tension for yourself and the child.

GET READY FOR MASSAGE

- Find a relaxed time that works for you both.
- Always ask the child's permission first, and respect their decision to receive, or not receive, nurturing touch.
- Give the child choice of music, oils and stories to be told – engage them in the activity.

DURING MASSAGE TIME

- During massage time – remember to smile, maintain eye contact and provide gentle touch.

- Be sure to use age appropriate language and explain what you are doing.
- Explain what they will feel, hear, smell and what they can expect from the massage.

AFTER MASSAGE TIME

- Ask how the child felt during and after the massage.
- Ask them to tell you about their favorite part of massage time.
- Ask for suggestions for next time.

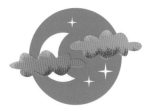

WHY PERMISSION IS IMPORTANT

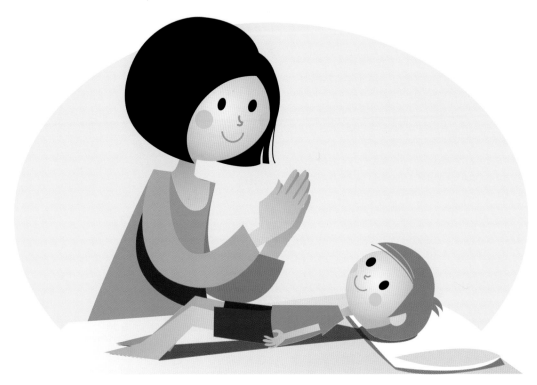

Children's massage is always linked with a "permission process". When used together, these practices help to reinforce respect for the child and begin to establish positive boundaries. Permission is really one of the most important elements in massage for children.

HOW TO ASK PERMISSION
- Rub your hands together to warm them.
- Show respect by looking at the child.
- Verbally ask if they would like to receive a massage.

We specifically ask permission prior to beginning massage for many reasons, including:

LETS THE CHILD KNOW WHAT IS ABOUT TO HAPPEN
Checking in with the child, rather than just assuming touch is okay, shows respect and gives them a choice to receive nurturing touch, or not.

Over time, the child begins to recognize this permission cue as "Massage Time", and will respond that they are ready for massage.

At no other time will you use this specific signal, or cue, to indicate what will happen next. This distinct permission process communicates your intention, and allows the child time to evaluate how they are feeling prior to responding.

GIVES YOU AN OPPORTUNITY TO CHECK-IN AND OBSERVE THEIR CUES

Touch is our first form of communication, so, it is natural to assume that communicating through touch enhances your ability to understand a child's needs and respond appropriately. Massage increases confidence and sensitivity to unique cues and forms of communication. By relaxing, taking your time and making eye contact, you can accurately observe a child's expression, and non-verbal language. Over time, you will become more attuned to their needs.

A SIMPLE PERMISSION PROCESS SUPPORTS HEALTHY TOUCH AND HELPS ESTABLISH GOOD BOUNDARIES

When we start asking permission to touch during the most formative years, we reinforce the concepts of good touch versus touch that may not be seen as good or positive touch. A young child will carry with them these healthy and strong boundaries around touch. Not only will they know the difference between healthy touch and touch which is considered detrimental, they will also trust themselves and know when to request nurturing touch.

ESTABLISHES RESPECT BETWEEN YOU AND THE CHILD, INSTILLING LIFELONG BENEFITS INCLUDING SELF-WORTH AND SELF-ESTEEM

Massage provides you with essential one-on-one time that will enhance your bonding, understanding and ability to nurture. When children receive attentive responses to their needs, they grow to become healthier and more secure in adulthood. Children who learn positive views of touch and receive nurturing touch are much more likely to grow into adults with healthy self esteem, a sense of their boundaries and increased self trust.

If a child is non-verbal, it might appear difficult to ask and receive permission. This isn't so. You should still ask permission in the same manner as you would with another child. However, instead of expecting a verbal "yes" or "no", look at the body language and cues. You will look for cues such as a relaxed, happy child who is smiling with wide open eyes that are looking at you. In general, if the child appears happy and doesn't run away, you likely have permission to begin.

The need for recognizing cues is why you cannot continue massage for a child who falls asleep, or begin when they are sleeping. You do not have permission. They have given no indication of their desire to receive massage. They can not tell you if it is uncomfortable or if they have any preferences.

In some cases, there are children who would greatly benefit from massage therapy, however, as it is a new activity, they may be unsure, scared or in pain. In such a circumstance, finding a way to gently introduce nurturing touch may be of great value. You might want to start with a professional giving the massage. In this way, the professional may be able to "break the ice" and teach you what works best.

NURTURING TOUCH FOR THE GROWING CHILD

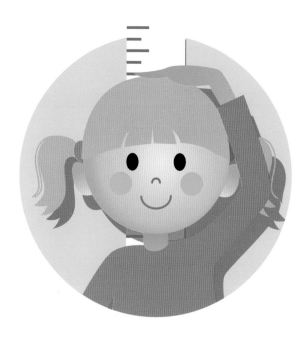

As a child grows and develops, they become more active and curious about the world around them.

Before they reach the age of 12, children are more tactile and kinesthetic, using their feelings more than sight or sound to gather information about the world. So, it is important to consider different ways to engage a child's interest in nurturing touch.

TODDLER (1 – 3 YEARS OLD)

You may know this first hand as you are currently raising, or have raised a toddler. Their attention span is short. The amount of time they may be interested in one activity is limited. With your massage time, it is suggested to include more songs, stories, rhymes and items (toys) that interest them.

With toddlers, it is sometimes easier to involve them in multiple short activities, as opposed to a long massage session. Play is extremely important and should be part of the massage time. Consider using puppets, or a child's favorite toy to make a connection. Massage stories are another great way to incorporate massage strokes into an age appropriate activity.

HELPFUL HINTS
- Limit the length of the massage time to adapt to a shorter attention span.
- Introduce a massage story and ask the child to add to the story.
- If the child has any soreness due to growing muscles, respect their request for the massage stroke to change, or end.

PRESCHOOL AGE (3 - 5 YEARS OLD)

Choose your words wisely. During this stage children often imitate words and actions. Be prepared to answer many "why" and "how" questions. Preschool aged children are very interested in playing "make believe" and have magical thinking. So, be creative and have fun! Another bonus, the preschooler's attention span is increasing. This may mean a longer massage time if your story is creative and interesting.

HELPFUL HINTS
- Use gentle massage strokes and support the child's joints.
- Adapt the pace and pressure of the strokes to help ease growing pains that usually occur just below the knee.
- Child may wish to learn about massage by providing massage for you or even a stuffed animal.

SCHOOL AGE (5 – 12 YEARS OLD)

The first important point here is that children at age 5 are quite different from children at age 12. During this changing stage, logical thinking begins, imagination broadens and the child's attention span grows. School age children are getting to know their peers and begin seeking independence from their parents. With this age group, it is important to remember that they enjoy feeling in control. During the 10 – 12 year age range, many children experience growth spurts and complain of growing pains.

HELPFUL HINTS
- Create a special time to check-in with the child and talk about their daily experiences.

- Offer massage in conjunction with sporting and extracurricular activities.
- Use massage as a way help the child to relax, easing stress and anxiety associated with academic pressures.

TEENAGE (12 – 18 YEARS OLD)

During the teen years, treating a teenager as a child is a big mistake. Even though they may be growing, and technically their brain is still developing, this young person seeks independence and respect. They generally speak much like an adult and should be approached with this type of comprehension in mind. Throughout these formative years, privacy is very important and should be respected. Many teens have concerns around body image and body changes due to puberty.

HELPFUL HINTS
- Massage may be helpful in promoting self esteem and self respect.
- Providing massage can often alleviate the discomfort associated with menstrual cramps.
- Try using gentle techniques to help balance hormones and aid in easing physical discomforts.

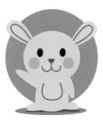

ALL ABOUT OIL FOR CHILDREN'S MASSAGE

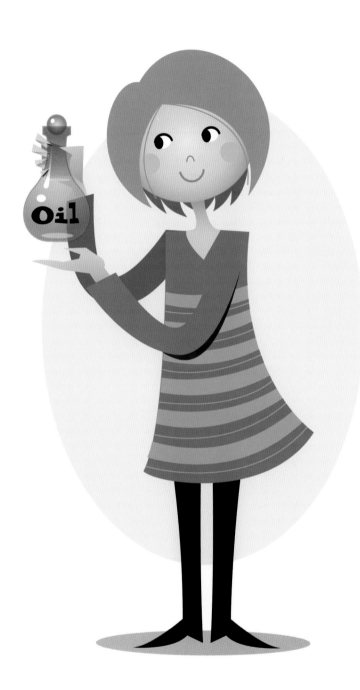

All oils put on the skin are absorbed into the skin to some extent and then move through the capillaries into the blood stream. A child's skin is still developing, and can absorb more easily than an adult's, so it is important to choose oil that is most suitable.

When choosing oil for massage, look for something that has been cold-pressed or expeller-pressed, as they last longer and have less potential to be contaminated with harmful compounds. Do not store oil in heat or under direct light. It is best to store oil in a cool dark place. Before using any stored oil, smell, and if necessary, taste the oil. Oil that has spoiled, or become rancid, will have an unusual smell and taste bitter. If unsure, throw the oil away. It's always best to proceed on the safer side when it comes to massage oil for children.

UNSCENTED, NATURAL, COLD-PRESSED, EDIBLE, FRUIT OR VEGETABLE OILS ARE RECOMMENDED FOR CHILDREN'S MASSAGE.

Some suggested oils for massage: **olive oil, grape seed, jojoba and sweet almond.**

HELPFUL HINTS
- When using oil, ensure the child is in a safe and

comfortable position. Their skin may become slippery during massage. They may slip and fall if standing, or roll off of an elevated surface.

- Oil may help your hands to glide more easily.
- Choose natural, edible, fragrance free oil.
- Choose fruit or vegetable based oils to help in cases where there is possible allergy to nut oils.
- Do not use synthetic oils such as mineral oil, as these may be harmful if ingested, may irritate the skin and if fragranced, may interfere with the bonding.
- Oil can help the child stay warm by retaining body temperature.

Do not use essential oils without the guidance of an experienced aromatherapist or healthcare provider. Essential oil used incorrectly may cause more harm than good.

SKIN PATCH TEST

Before using any oil, it is a good idea to perform a simple patch test to ensure the child does not have any immediate allergic reaction to the oil chosen. Some children have allergies to nut based and wheat based oils.

To perform a simple patch test, apply a small amount of oil to the child's skin at least thirty minutes prior to massage to allow enough time for a severe reaction to present itself. This will check for immediate hypersensitivity reactions.

Choose a location on the body that the child cannot easily reach, or irritate.

Observe the skin and notice if any blotches or discolorations appear. If there is any sign of an allergic reaction, do not use the oil.

If there is no reaction to the oil, you may wish to proceed with the massage.

If the child is having trouble over time with skin reactions, you may want to perform a more sophisticated patch test, or have this done by an allergist. This tests for delayed hypersensitivity, which is a common way for the body to react to things on the skin. For instance, Posion Ivy does not cause an immediate reaction, but has a delayed hypersensitivity reaction that is only evident after 48-72 hours. It is mediated by a different part of the immune system. In this more sophisticated patch testing, the oil or suspected substance is placed on the skin and held in place by a band aid or something similar, and then reaction is looked for after 72 hours.

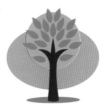

DRAPING AND PRIVACY DURING MASSAGE

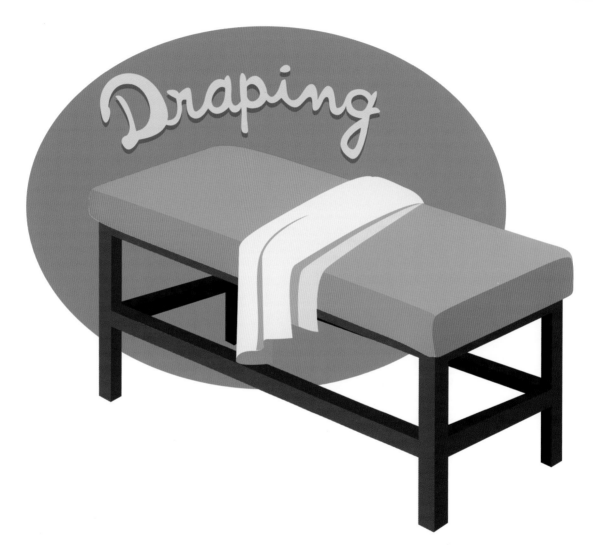

It is important to maintain privacy at all times. Misunderstandings may occur if a child's privacy has been compromised.

Ensuring proper privacy and draping techniques may help to avoid this situation. Draping is the method of covering the body with a towel or sheet, if you are not actively massaging those areas. With children, draping should be more conservative and modest than standard adult massage.

HELPFUL HINTS

- Never let the child dress or undress in front of you. As a parent, this rule may be slightly different, as you may assist your child if they are unable to change their clothing on their own.
- Children may keep any or all of their clothing on during massage.
- Never place your hands under clothing if your hands would then not be seen by the child.
- Using age appropriate language, explain draping to the child. Make sure they understand they will not be exposed unnecessarily.
- With toddlers, it is advised to ask them to keep their underclothes on. Toddlers playing peek-a-boo with your sheets is common practice, and may lead to unnecessary exposure if they remove their undergarments.
- A parent may find their child welcomes touch on their back underneath their clothing. This may be provided, so long as by the parent of the child in a safe and nurturing manner. The child needs to give permission for this type of touch.
- Do not expose more of the child's body than absolutely necessary. Expose only the region you are currently working on.
- At any time a child displays any feelings of discomfort with any exposure, you should cover this area immediately.

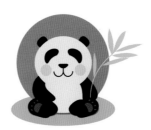

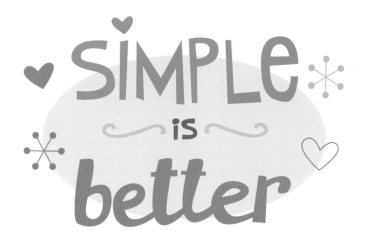

Children's massage does not have to be complicated, aggressive or deep to be effective. Sometimes, simple is better for the body and mind.

When we over complicate our massage time, it may take more work for the child to process all of the sensory information received.

The techniques appearing here may be used to provide a full body massage for a child. You would simply use gentle pressure, and adapt the size and shape of the strokes to best fit the region on which you are working. Other strokes you may add include "hugs" (gentle compressions with warmed palms of your hand gently "hugging" the child's body area), "rain" (light finger tapping) and "thunder" (gentle percussion with a cupped hand).

CHILDREN'S MASSAGE STROKES | HOW TO
Begin with Nurturing Touch and then follow with the remaining strokes on each area of the body where the child welcomes touch.

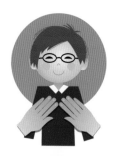

NURTURING TOUCH

Loving and still, rest your hands and introduce your touch to the area where you will begin.

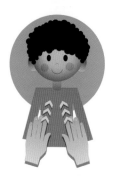

GENTLE WARMING GLIDE

With warm palms, gently stroke the body in long fluid movements toward the heart.

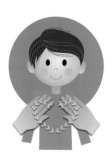

OPEN HEART

Draw "Heart" shapes on the area you are working. Vary the size of the hearts from little to big, depending on the size of the area.

CROSS MY HEART

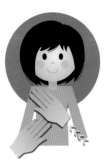

On the back, chest and other larger areas you may also draw "X's" with you finger pads and palms. By drawing an "X" you are intentionally crossing the midline of the body further encouraging left brain, right brain functioning.

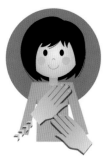

CRISS-CROSS

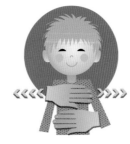

Alternating hands, glide them back and forth across the area you are working on.

GENTLE SOOTHING GLIDE

With warm palms, gently stroke the body area in a long fluid motion in the direction away from the heart. This gliding stroke let's the child know we have finished with this area.

SOME CONSIDERATIONS

Some children may not prefer the name of the stroke "open heart" which is described in the massage routine above. Feel free to use your creativity and change it.

Some good suggestions include baseballs, clouds, circles, footballs and hockey pucks. You can even allow the child to help you make up a similar shaped massage stroke of their own.

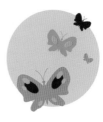

ADDRESSING COMMON CHILDHOOD DISCOMFORTS

ABDOMINAL MASSAGE FOR CONSTIPATION, GAS AND TUMMY ACHES

A common complaint of many children, is upset tummies. Not only due to eating too much ice cream and candy, but other times, the child may experience discomfort from excess gas, constipation, or even stress. Abdominal massage has proven very effective in helping with elimination and relief.

CHILDREN'S MASSAGE STROKES | ABDOMINAL MASSAGE HOW TO

The techniques below are described with the child laying on their back looking at you.
They may be performed in other positions, but it is imperative that the strokes follow the correct direction.

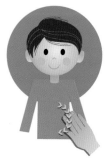

MOON

With your right hand, trace a half circle (moon shape) on child's tummy from 12 o'clock - 6 o'clock.

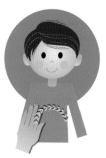

RAINBOW

Draw a big rainbow, starting on child's right side (your left) draw to child's left side (your right) REMEMBER: clockwise motion only.

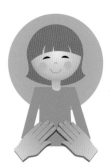

NURTURING TOUCH

Loving and still, rest your warm palms on the tummy.

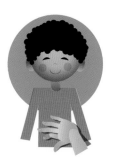

STARS

Using the pads of your finger tips, gently march across child's tummy from child's right side to child's left side in a rainbow shape.

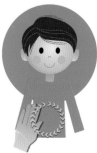

SUN

Place left hand on child's tummy and make a large clockwise circle.

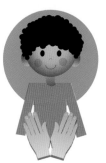

SOOTHING STROKE

Gently stroke down the tummy to signal the end of this massage.

BENEFITS OF MASSAGE FOR CONSTIPATION, GAS AND TUMMY ACHES

- Improves functioning of the gastrointestinal tract
- Increases fluid in the gastrointestinal tract and causes movement.
- Provides manual stimulation and assists in the expulsion of waste.

HELPFUL HINTS

- When making circular strokes on the abdominal area, they should always follow the direction of the child's digestive tract. For the vast majority, this is a clockwise direction moving from the child's right side to left side.
- Wait approximately 30 minutes after the child has eaten to provide massage therapy techniques on the abdomen.
- Provide massage techniques on the soft areas of the child's abdomen, from the bottom of their rib cage down. Do not put any pressure on the Xyphoid process, the cartilaginous section at the lower end of the sternum, which is not attached to any ribs and gradually hardens during adult life.
- Do not press too firmly or deeply.
- If the child asks you to stop, or shows sign of discomfort, stop providing massage.
- Use a simple rhyme to help keep the child's interest.

THE SUN IS OUT ALL DAY
THE MOON COMES OUT AT NIGHT
RAINBOWS MAKE ME HAPPY
& THE STARS ARE SPARKLY BRIGHT

MASSAGE FOR CONGESTION

Congestion is a common concern throughout childhood. Whether the child is getting over a cold, or suffers from allergies, massage therapy may be very helpful in eliminating some symptoms and easing discomfort. Massage should not be performed if the child is unwell, has a fever, or any type of infection except under the guidance of the child's healthcare provider, or other professional who is part of the child's healthcare team. With proper guidance, you may be able to provide massage and help play a nurturing role in the child's care.

BENEFITS OF MASSAGE FOR CONGESTION

- May help to relax tight muscles around the ribcage.
- Cupped hand percussion may loosen mucus and secretions.
- Air intake may be increased following massage therapy.
- Can decrease anxiety and stress hormones (cortisol and norepinephrine levels).
- Improves lung capacity and pulmonary functions.
- Aids in opening sinus passages.
- Increases immunity.
- Provides opportunity for relaxation.

HELPFUL HINTS AND ADAPTATIONS

- Position child at 45° angle if possible (laying on their back, use pillows for support behind upper torso).
- Use moderate pressure and smooth strokes.
- Provide massage over the entire body, paying special attention to the back, muscles next to spinal column, chest and ribcage area.
- Provide "cross my heart" stroke on the chest and back.

- Spend a few extra moments massaging the back, paying close attention to the muscles on the sides of the spinal column.
- May gently apply cupped hand percussion on the back, do not apply pressure directly on the spine

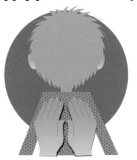

- Provide massage over the areas of the body where the child welcomes massage, while at the same time, respecting vulnerable "no-touch" areas. Do not provide massage on the areas undergarments would cover. These areas include the genitals, buttocks, and chest close to the nipple region. Any area that causes the child to feel uncomfortable would be a "no-touch" area. It is important that massage is used as a safe, respectful and nurturing shared activity.
- Paying special attention to face, glide down the sides of child's nose, stopping just to the side of the nostrils for a short finger press (do not use too much pressure); then glide across the cheeks to the outside of the face, and up the sides of the face around the eyes, back to the middle of the forehead.

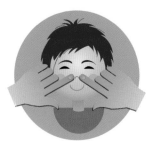

- Provide circular strokes on cheeks.

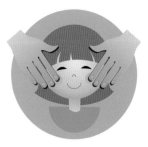

- Provide gentle pressure on eyebrow pressure points.

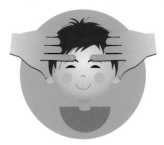

MASSAGE FOR GROWING PAINS

Many children experience growing pains. Some complain of aches in their lower limbs, while others may wake up crying in the middle of the night. Often times we think of growing pains occurring during school age. However, due to their rapid growth rate, toddlers may also experience significant growing pains.

BENEFITS OF MASSAGE FOR GROWING PAINS
- Promotes relaxation.
- Soothes muscle tension and may calm muscle spasms.
- Assists in relief of pain and discomfort.
- Improves circulation.
- May support lengthening of soft tissues.
- May aid in increased endorphin release.

HELPFUL HINTS AND ADAPTATIONS

- Gently hug (gently cup the muscle in between your two palms) the calf muscles, as if kneading dough; focus on the upper muscle area just below the knee.

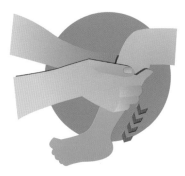

- Follow hugging by rolling down the calf muscles as if you are rolling dough.
- When hugging and rolling, do not put any pressure on the bones on front of the calves.
- Repeat hugging 3 times, followed by rolling 3 times.
- Repeat all techniques on other leg.
- If a muscle spasm begins, pause – change strokes or position.

MASSAGE FOR HEADACHES

Childhood headaches are unfortunately quite common. If you are concerned about a child's complaints of headaches, a visit to a healthcare provider may be recommended. Headaches and migraines are typically uncommon before the age of four, but all types of headaches seem to increase as children get older. Many children have an enormous amount of peer, family and academic pressure which may contribute to their headaches.

BENEFITS OF MASSAGE FOR HEADACHES

- Provides opportunity for relaxation.
- Aids in stress relief.
- Assists in relief of muscle tension.
- May increase endorphins (our body's natural pain killers).

HELPFUL HINTS AND ADAPTATIONS

- Provide massage for the entire body while respecting "no-touch" areas, paying special attention to the upper back, shoulders, neck and head (scalp).
- Use "cross my heart" stroke on back.

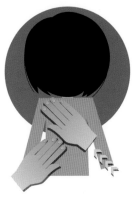

- Gently place both hands and shoulders and "hug" the shoulders simultaneously.

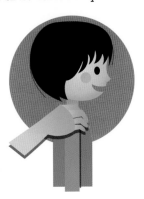

- Gently massage "headache point", located on the back of the hand, in the webbing where the thumb and index finger meet.

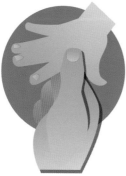

- Use gentle holding on the "1, 2, 3" pressure points in the eyebrow area.

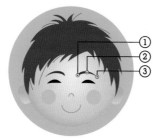

- Use gentle holding on the base of the head.

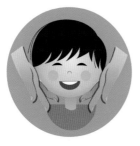

MASSAGE FOR SLEEPING DIFFICULTIES

Childhood sleeping difficulties are quite common and may range from a child having difficulty falling asleep to not sleeping through the night. Some children experience difficulties due to built up tension and stress, while others may have "separation anxiety" and emotional challenges with sleeping. A good night's sleep, however, is very important, as this is when the largest percentage of growth takes place.

BENEFITS OF MASSAGE FOR SLEEPING DIFFICULTIES

- Provides an opportunity to relax and decrease anxiety.
- May decrease the length of time it takes to fall asleep.
- Promotes the increase of delta waves (those linked with deep restorative sleep).
- May aid in reduction of cortisol (stress hormone).
- May increase serotonin (feel good, happy and relaxing hormone).
- Helps the child sleep deeper and for longer periods of time.
- If given by parent(s), may provide essential bonding time, decrease separation anxiety, and become an essential part of a nurturing bedtime routine.

ADAPTATIONS

- Strokes should be slow, rhythmic and move away from the heart.
- Consider using a massage story in place of a bedtime story.
- If teeth grinding is a problem, pay special attention to the jaw, chin, head and neck.

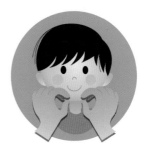

- Stroke on the center forehead between the eyes, down towards the tip of the nose.

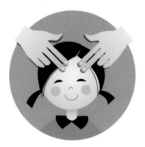

MASSAGE FOR STRESS AND TENSION

There are many causes of stress in a child's life. These may include a traumatic event, accident or injury to someone they love, being hurt in a violent manner, bullies, peer pressure, academic anxiety, divorce, parental military service deployment, moving, and death of a family pet can cause tension and anxiety. For teens, peer pressure, wondering if someone thinks you're attractive, not having enough privacy, moving to a new school, not having enough money or having a teacher who doesn't like you can equal unimaginable stress.

BENEFITS OF MASSAGE FOR STRESS AND TENSION

- Provides opportunity to soothe, relax and calm.
- Aids in decrease of anxiety.
- May improve accompanying conditions such as headaches and stomach aches.

ADAPTATIONS

- Provide massage over entire body while respecting "no-touch" areas, paying special attention to back, shoulders, neck and head.

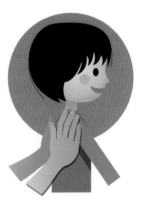

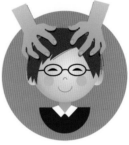

- Ensure the child feels in control during the massage.
- Consider positioning the child sitting up and asking them to keep all clothes on.
- Be mindful of emotional sensitivity in chest area.
- Provide massage on hands and feet.
- Stroke down back to calm nervous system.

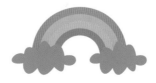

STORIES, SONGS/MUSIC, RHYMES AND MOVEMENT GAMES

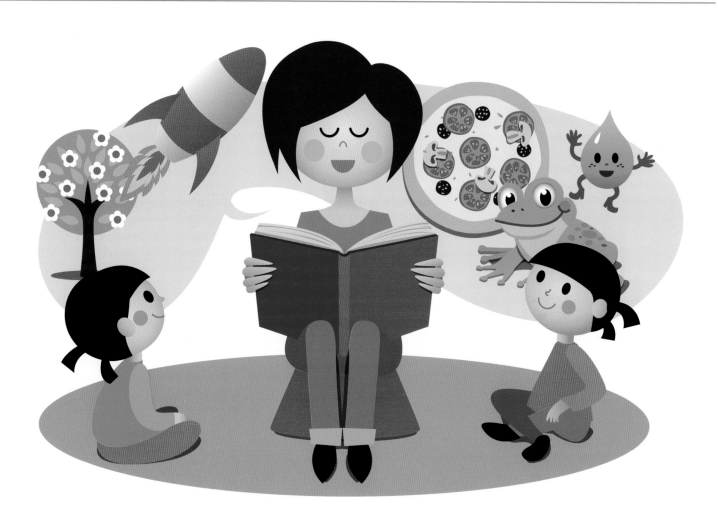

Using child friendly and age appropriate stories, songs, rhymes and movement games, can help to further strengthen your connection with the child both verbally and non-verbally.

Reading and reciting stories to a child is one of the best ways to boost their language and comprehension skills. When you are selecting your stories, ensure they are age-appropriate, have a fairly simple story line, and pleasant ending. It is often easiest to limit nurturing touch which accompanies storytelling to massage on the back. It would best serve the massage experience to avoid stories which may be frightening or scary.

Classic stories often provide familiarity and optimal storytelling opportunities. However, stories may be based on a favorite character, subject or designed specifically for massage time.

SONGS & MUSIC

Children of all ages may benefit from the use of auditory stimulation and rhythm in conjunction with touch therapy. It is important when choosing music selections, specific emphasis is placed on choosing selections that are developmentally appropriate.

You can provide a sensory rich environment by providing musical stimulation in a variety of ways. Beginning about age 2, children start trying to repeat back musical phrases, show physical responses to music and can clearly differentiate between tempos and rhythms.

Toddlers love to explore music through body movements. To create the most sensory rich environment, provide opportunity for dancing and movement. For example, if you are singing about flowers, give the child a flower and let them wave it about as they sing, or try using a massage story that goes along with this theme, and plant a garden on the child's back.

For young children, consider simple, classic songs such as "You Are My Sunshine", "The Ants Go Marching", "The Itsy Bitsy Spider", "Head, Shoulders, Knees and Toes" and "Happy and You Know It".

Considering older children, incorporate music that is age-appropriate and pleasing to the child. Let the child select their listening pleasure. Bare in mind, we may not feel that their selection is appropriate for massage, as it is loud or very upbeat. However, if the child enjoys the tune, and it causes them to be happy and relaxed, this is the perfect choice. Especially be considerate of this when providing massage for an adolescent. Often times, their music choices are not the same as ours. As long as the song does not have a negative message, this is absolutely fine when it comes to massage time.

RHYMES

Using short, simple and fun rhymes are another great way to incorporate language, connection and enhance verbal abilities. By using an engaging rhyme, you may also cause the child to become more interested in the massage time together and thus lengthen the experience.

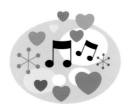

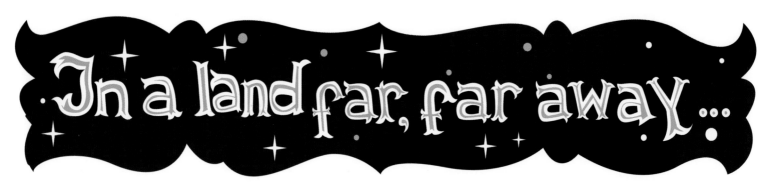

In a land far, far away ➡ Rest your warmed palms on back

Over mountains and streams ➡ Press softly and gently all over the back

There is a lovely place created entirely in our dreams ➡ Move hands across back in swirling motion

Where the sun is out all day ➡ Draw a big, round sun on back

And the moon comes out at night ➡ Draw half moon on back with right hand

Colorful rainbows make me happy ➡ Draw big rainbow (upside down U) on back alternating hands

And stars are sparkly bright ➡ Walk fingertips all over back

Fluffy clouds are seen way up high ➡ Gently press your palms at top of back

And sprinkling raindrops fall from the sky ➡ Press fingertips on back moving from upper back to lower

There is wind and laughter ➡ Move hands in swirly motion all over the back

And chilly weather too ...brrr! ➡ Wiggle fingertips on back

Sometimes the sky turns to gray from blue ➡ Continue wiggling motion on back

Lightening is seen ➡ Move hands across back – "Criss-Cross"

And thunder is heard → Gently apply percussion with cupped hands

Don't worry yourself → Bring hands still and rest them on the back

Its not much louder than a bird → Hands continue to rest on back

In the winter it gets colder and colder still

Soft fluffy flakes fall → Move hands gently, and press palms on back

And cover every hill → Sprinkle the back with light fingertips

Soon we realize the land is coated in white → Make swirly motions on the back

Bringing the calm as still as night → Rest hands on shoulders

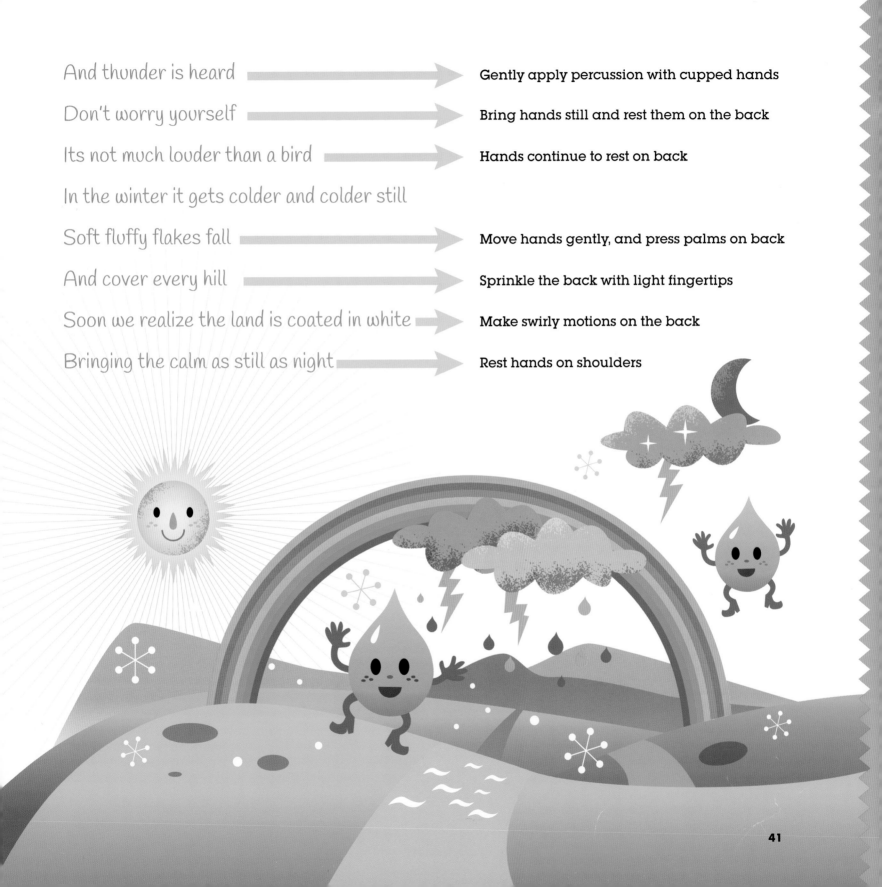

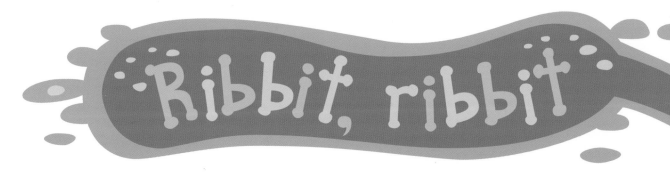

Start with hands resting on shoulders

Looking out far and beyond —→ Use palms and "hop" them gently all over the back

We see a frog hopping, hopping —→ Continue with hopping motion

Above an icy pond —→ Press palms flat on back and wiggle them back and forth

He ribbits, and shivers —→ Hop the palms back up to the shoulders

And hops way up high —→ Rest hands on shoulders

Until he almost reaches the sky —→ Leave hands resting

Taking his spot on the mossy mound —→ Gently hug each shoulder

He wiggles into place

Soon the warm sun rose in the west —→ Draw a big, round sun on the back

Doing all it can to melt the rest —→ Continue circular motions

The ice drips away —→ Using finger tips, comb down the back

And snow melts too —→ Continue with combing motion

The gloomy sky soon turns from gray to blue	Using finger tips, comb down the back
The frogs hop away	Make hopping motions all over the back
Finding a lilypad new	Softly rest hands on shoulders
Children begin to play	Move hands all over back in wiggly motions
And no one is sad	Continue movements
Everyone is happy with smiles that glow	Draw big smiles on back ("U" Shapes)
Enjoying the warm spring	Move hands to low back
Before the next winter's snow	Bring hands straight up and sweep over the shoulders
	Continue this sweeping motion three times

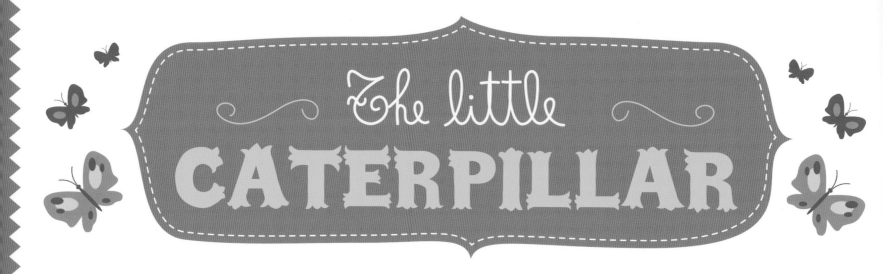

The little CATERPILLAR

The Little Caterpillar lies down for a rest ⟹ Have child lay down on tummy, sitting on heels

Sleeping soundly and dreaming ⟹ Draw warm sunbeams

The sun is shining ⟹ Sweep your hands in a big circle shape

There is a gentle breeze ⟹ Gently sweep hands back & forth

The wind gets stronger ⟹ Swirl both hands around the back

Even stronger – a storm is coming! ⟹ Move both hands back & forth across the back

It starts to rain ⟹ Tap fingers all over the back

Then it begins to pour down ⟹ Tap fingers with slightly more pressure

Ooh! Lightening! ⟹ Zig-zag your hands down the back

And thunder too! ....➔ Cup your hands and tap the palms over the back (avoiding spine). Cupped hands make a clapping sound

Then the rain slows down ....➔ Lightly tap fingers all over the back

The sun comes out & warms the ....➔ Sweep your hands in a big circle shape
Caterpillar who has now become a
beautiful butterfly

The butterfly wakes and stretches his ....➔ Move your hands from middle of child's back down
wings each arm and spread arms open to imitate flying
butterfly wings

Happy to be warmed by the sun, and flies
away

Not all massage stories need to rhyme. Some stories can
simply be created on the spot using your creativity and
the child's imagination.
The idea is to relax, ask permission, and most
importantly, have fun!

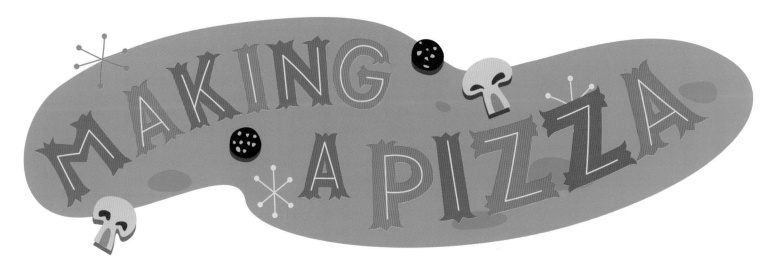

Do you think we should make a pizza?
Let's start by pressing flour all over our
table before we roll out the dough ➡ **Lightly glide down the back and begin to lightly press all over the back**

Now we're ready to knead the dough ➡ **Glide your hands up to the shoulder and gently knead the shoulders**

Let's begin to roll out the dough in a
great big circle ➡ **Move hands in a big circle covering the entire back**

Let's go ahead and add some tomato
sauce ➡ **Gently glide your hands back and forth across the back**

Now we need to sprinkle on some cheese ➡ **Lightly tap fingers all over back**

Let's start adding the toppings, how
about some pepperoni first? ➡ **Draw small circles all over the back**

And maybe some mushrooms? ➡ **Draw small circles all over the back**

Let's try some tomatoes → Using soft cupped hands, place them and move them in a circular motion on the back

And a little more cheese → Lightly tap fingers all over back

Now we just wait for a pizza to get nice and hot → Move your hands in a circular motion a few times

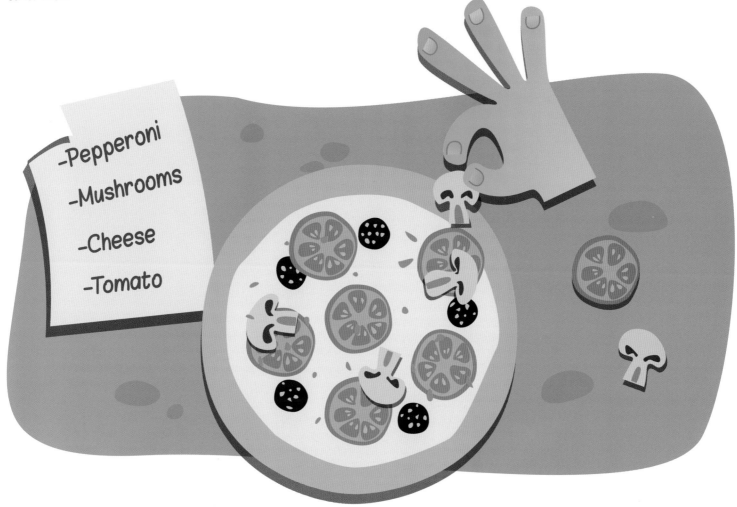

-Pepperoni
-Mushrooms
-Cheese
-Tomato

When making a pizza, planting a garden, or baking cookies – it's a great idea to ask the children what they would like to add.

Over time, they will learn the types of touch they prefer, and request it in the form of rain, snow and chocolate chips!

FOUR SEASONS RHYME

Place hands on back gently resting

Rain is falling down, splish ⟶ Move fingertips, walking down back from shoulders to high waist

Rain is falling down, splash ⟶ Bring hands back to shoulders . . .repeat moving your fingertips, walking down back from shoulders to high waist

Pitter patter, pitter patter ⟶ Move fingertips in rhythmic dancing "side-to-side" movement on lower back

Rain is falling down, splish ⟶ Move fingertips, walking down back from shoulders to high waist

Rain is falling down, splash ⟶ Bring hands back to shoulders . . .repeat moving your fingertips, walking down back from shoulders to high waist

Sun is peeking out, peek! ⟶ Bring your hands back to the shoulders and rest them on both shoulders. Gently hug one shoulder

Sun is peeking out, peek! ⟶ Gently hug the other shoulder

Peeking here, peeking there ⟶ Gently hug both shoulders simultaneously

Sun is peeking out, peek! ⟶ Make big, warm circles with your two palms on the child's back

Snow is Falling Down, shh!	→ Gently press full palms lightly on child's back starting at shoulders
Snow is Falling Down, shh!	→ Moving down to mid back
Slowly, slowly, very slowly	→ Now moving palms slowly up and down entire back
Snow is Falling Down, shh!	→ Continue these gentle presses until you once again reach the shoulder
All is quiet and still	→ Rest your hands gently and still on the shoulders

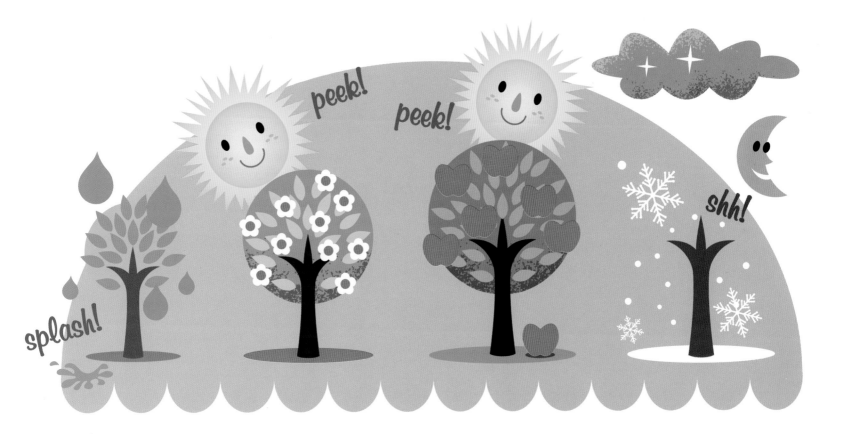

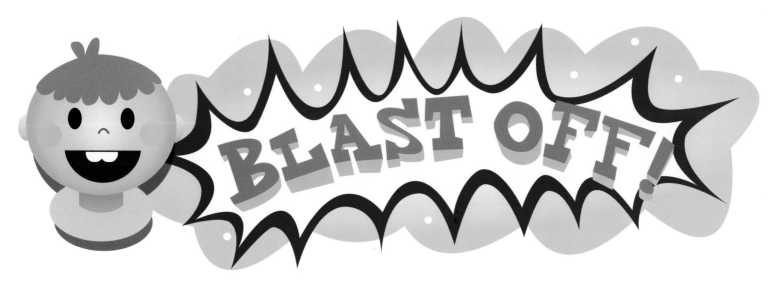

Place hands on back gently resting

I am a little rocket → Move palms in a warm circular motion on child's back

Standing on the ground → Glide palms down from shoulders to waist three times

Waiting quietly → Keep warmed palms still on the mid-waist

Without a sound → Hold perfectly still

Light the fuse down below → Swirl hands on mid-waist

Ready for blast off → Make swirl movements all over the back and bring them back to mid-waist

Here we go → Bring warmed palms up the back from mid-waist to shoulders three to five times

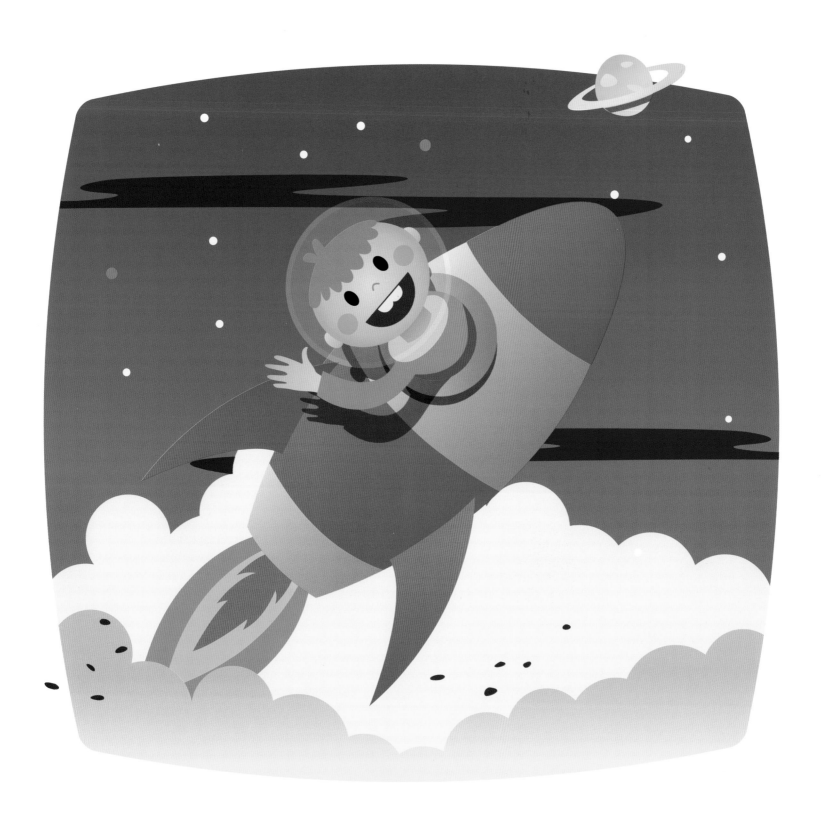

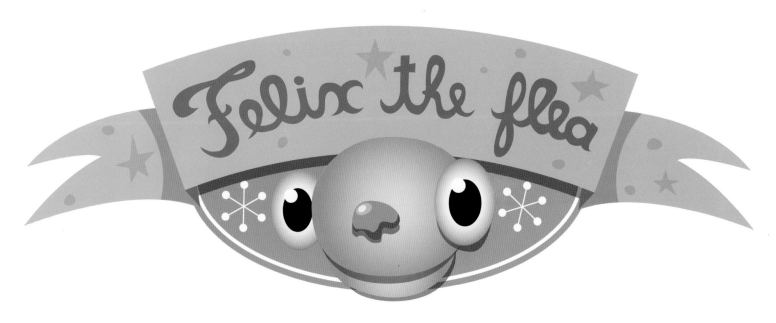

Place hands on back gently resting

On my head there is a flea ⋯⋯⋯⋯ Allow hands to sit on head

Starting to climb down on me ⋯⋯⋯⋯ Move hands in circular motions on head

Moving from where my hair grows ⋯⋯⋯ Move hands gently from head down neck

Soon he will pass my nose ⋯⋯⋯⋯ Continue to shoulders

Over my shoulders, and down my back ⋯⋯ Walk with gentle fingertips from shoulders starting down the back

Felix the Flea acts like a maniac ⋯⋯ Make slow, swirly movements all over the back and bring them back to mid-waist

Faster and faster he goes ⋯⋯⋯⋯ Increase speed of swirling movements

Where he stops, I don't know ⟶ Bring warmed palms to mid-back and rest

Past my belly and down to my waist ⟶ Gently move with fingertips down back to waist

There he sits without haste ⟶ Rest palms on waist

Taking a nap for all to see ⟶ Provide gentle hugs on waist and low back

No one is happier than Felix the Flea ⟶ Bring hands still

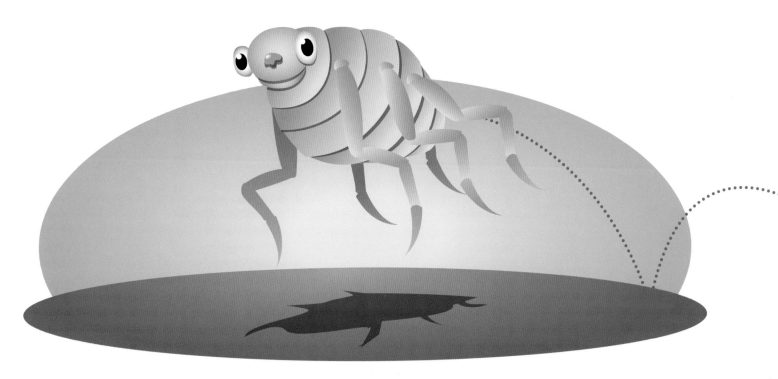

Movement & Games: During your massage time, consider incorporating simple movement activities and games to make the time together more enjoyable and provide the richest sensory experience.

Head, shoulders, knees & toes is an example of using movement, music/singing and tactile input to create a sensory rich experience.

WHEN NOT TO MASSAGE

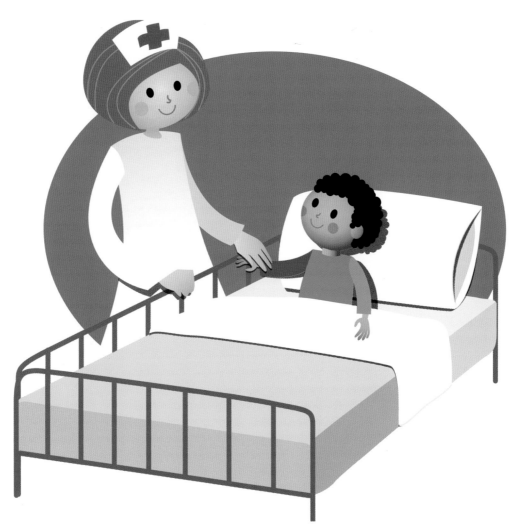

The massage and touch therapy suggestions described herein are to be used for children who are generally healthy and well.

If a child has any specific healthcare related conditions/diagnosis, pediatric massage for special healthcare needs may be required. Additionally, in these special situations, you may also wish to consult a child's healthcare provider before beginning massage.

There are times when massage is not recommended. Times when massage is completely off-limits are known as contraindications. Of course, the first thing to keep in mind is, massage is only performed with the child's permission to help encourage appropriate boundaries, safety and clarity of healthy touch. We also practice precaution, and although in some cases massage therapy is off-limits, we may be able to practice nurturing touch while following caution.

SOME CONSIDERATIONS

- Always follow the guidance of the healthcare provider.
- Always ask the child's permission to receive touch.
- Adjust and adapt the massage strokes for the comfort and care of the child.
- Always consider both the child's medical and emotional needs. Begin massage where there is the most access for skin-to-skin contact (for example, on the hands and feet).
- Use care and caution in areas where the child may have experienced pain.
- Always begin with Nurturing Touch.
- When culturally appropriate, always begin the massage with eye contact, especially with a child who may have hearing impairments.
- Always continue speaking throughout massage, especially with a child who may have visual impairments.

CONTRAINDICATIONS FOR CHILDREN'S MASSAGE

- Any special healthcare condition or diagnosis you do not understand (seek healthcare guidance).
- Cardiac conditions (heart conditions).

- Circulatory conditions.
- Respiratory distress or failure.
- Fever (above 100.5°).
- Pertussis, Influenza or active Tuberculosis.
- Acute, unstable or advanced conditions of the kidney or liver.
- Inflammation and Edema.
- Very High Blood Pressure.
- Swollen lymph nodes or infection of any kind.
- Hernia or abdominal distention.
- Osteoporosis, Brittle bones or Broken bones.
- Varicose Veins.
- Open wounds, sores or lesions (wet, sticky, not yours – don't touch it).
- Deep Vein Thrombosis, blood clots or serious blood conditions.
- Massage that causes pain.
- Skin Conditions or disorders which may be contagious or cause inflammation (fungus, rashes, herpes).
- Recent immunization/vaccination (wait 72 hours).
- Recent accident or injury.

CAUTIONARY SITES

Cautionary sites are areas of the body where you should practice additional caution, so as not to do harm.

Providing massage for a prolonged length of time, or with too much pressure, in these cautionary areas may cause damage to areas underneath the skin's surface.

AREAS TO PRACTICE CAUTION, USE LIGHTER PRESSURE OR AVOID, INCLUDE:

- "No-touch" areas - these areas include the genitals, buttocks, and chest close to the nipple region.

Any area that causes the child to feel uncomfortable would be a "no-touch" area.

- Back of elbow and inner elbow.
- Back of the knee.
- Eyes.
- Inner upper arm.
- Inner upper leg and groin.
- Joints.
- Mid-back near kidneys.
- Naval.
- Neck and throat.
- Spine and bony areas.
- Under arm.
- Xyphoid process.

HOSPITALIZED CHILDREN AND CHILDREN WITH VARIOUS SPECIAL HEALTHCARE NEEDS

It would be unfair to limit touch therapy and nurturing touch to only those children who we label as "healthy". Many children are quite appropriate for nurturing touch, and even pediatric massage.

However, it is extremely important that caution is followed when we are considering using this therapy with children who have been hospitalized, or require different care.

Prior to considering nurturing touch or massage for children who have special healthcare considerations, you should consult the child's healthcare provider. Never provide massage for a child that may have a pre-existing healthcare condition without first seeking guidance from the healthcare provider. Without guidance, you may jeopardize the child's condition, and actually do more harm than good.

When providing touch therapy for children who have, or are currently receiving any type of medical intervention, we must be mindful of those areas where they may have felt uncomfortable touch. Practice care and caution in these areas, consider adapting touch therapy to meet the needs of the child and introduce touch slowly.

As much as research indicates that pediatric massage can be very beneficial for children with a variety of healthcare needs, specific massage techniques and routines are utilized with children who have a variety of conditions and diagnoses. These adaptations are not included within this book. Specialized techniques should be performed by a qualified pediatric massage therapist, or shared with parents by a certified pediatric massage therapist. It is not safe to "dabble" in this area.

Always practice with safety and concern, to best care for children!

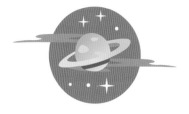

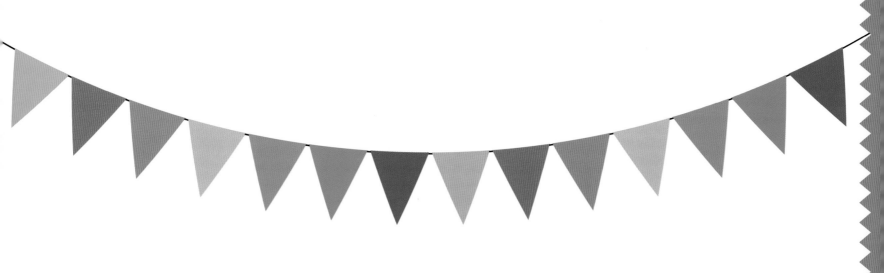

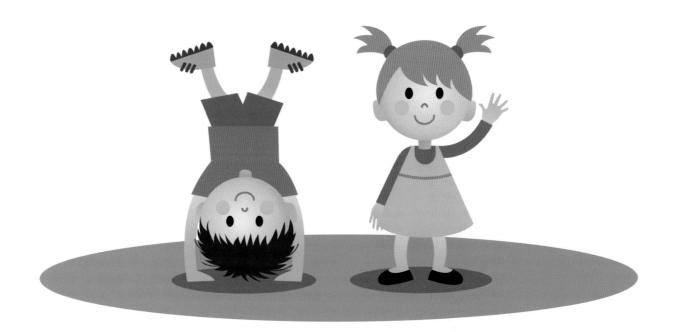

INDEX